The Fit and Healthy Mediterranean Recipe Collection

Super Simple Delicious Recipes

Affordable For Beginners

Alison Russell

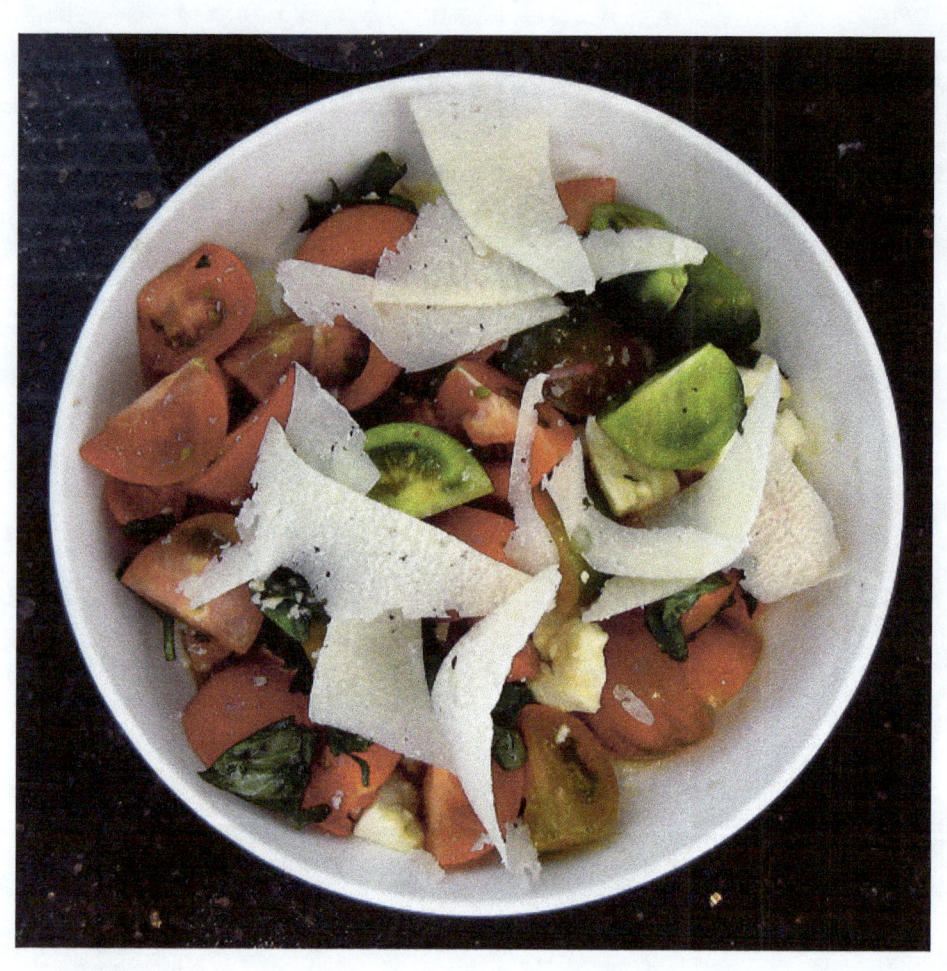

© **Copyright 2020 - All rights reserved.**

The content contained within this book may not be reproduced, duplicated or transmitted without direct written permission from the author or the publisher.

Under no circumstances will any blame or legal responsibility be held against the publisher, or author, for any damages, reparation, or monetary loss due to the information contained within this book. Either directly or indirectly.

Legal Notice:

This book is copyright protected. This book is only for personal use. You cannot amend, distribute, sell, use, quote or paraphrase any part, or the content within this book, without the consent of the author or publisher.

Disclaimer Notice:

Please note the information contained within this document is for educational and entertainment purposes only. All effort has been executed to present accurate, up to date, and reliable, complete information. No warranties of any kind are declared or implied. Readers acknowledge that the author is not engaging in the rendering of legal, financial, medical or professional advice. The content within this book has been derived from various sources. Please consult a licensed professional before attempting any techniques outlined in this book.

By reading this document, the reader agrees that under no circumstances is the author responsible for any losses, direct or indirect, which are incurred as a result of the use of information contained within this document, including, but not limited to, — errors, omissions, or inaccuracies.

Table of contents

Breakfast 8
   Oatmeal Banana Pancakes With Walnuts 9
   Creamy Oats, Greens and Blueberry Smoothie 12
   Carrot and Bran Mini Muffins 13
   French toast 16
   Jolene's Green Juice 18
   Chocolate Banana Smoothie 20
   Mediterranean Frittata 21
   Mediterranean Eggs 23
   Southwest Tofu Scramble 26
   Mediterranean Breakfast Salad 28
Lunch 30
   Easy Tuna Patties 31
   Fish Tacos 34
   Blackened Salmon Fillets 36
   Brown Butter Perch 38
   Almond Crust Chicken 40
   Mushroom Cheese Salad 43
   Shrimp Sandwiches 45
   Asparagus Salad 47

Mushrooms and Cheese Spread 50

Italian Baked Beans 52

Cannellini Bean Lettuce Wraps 54

Israeli Eggplant, Chickpea, and Mint Sauté 57

Minestrone Chickpeas and Macaroni Casserole 60

Mediterranean Lentils and Rice 62

Polenta with Sautéed Chard and Fried Eggs 65

Dinner 67

Simple Beef Sirloin Roast 68

Garlicky Pork Tenderloin 70

Greek Lamb Chops 73

Delicious Cauliflower Rice 74

Grilled Eggplant 76

Flavorful Roasted Vegetables 78

Healthy Carrot Salad 81

Beetroot & Carrot Salad 83

Dill Chutney Salmon 84

Garlic-Butter Parmesan Salmon and Asparagus 86

Lemon Rosemary Roasted Branzino 88

Grilled Lemon Pesto Salmon 90

Steamed Trout with Lemon Herb Crust 91

Desserts 93
    Crème Caramel 94
    Galaktoboureko 96
    Kourabiedes Almond Cookies 98
    Ekmek Kataifi 100
    Revani Syrup Cake 103
    Almonds and Oats Pudding 105
    Milk Chocolate Peanut Butter 107
    Cups 107

Breakfast

Oatmeal Banana Pancakes With Walnuts

Preparation Time: 15 minutes

Cooking Time: 5 minutes

Servings: 8 pancakes

Ingredients:

- 1 finely diced firm banana
- 1 c. whole wheat pancake mix
- 1/8 c. chopped walnuts
- 1/4 c. old-fashioned oats

Directions:

1. Make the pancake according to the directions on the package.
2. Add walnuts, oats, and chopped banana.
3. Coat a griddle with cooking spray. Attach about 1/4 cup of the pancake batter onto the griddle when hot.
4. Turn pancake over when bubbles form on top. Cook until golden brown.
5. Serve immediately.

Nutrition:

Calories: 155

Fat: 4 g

Carbs: 28 g

Protein: 7 g

Sodium: 10%

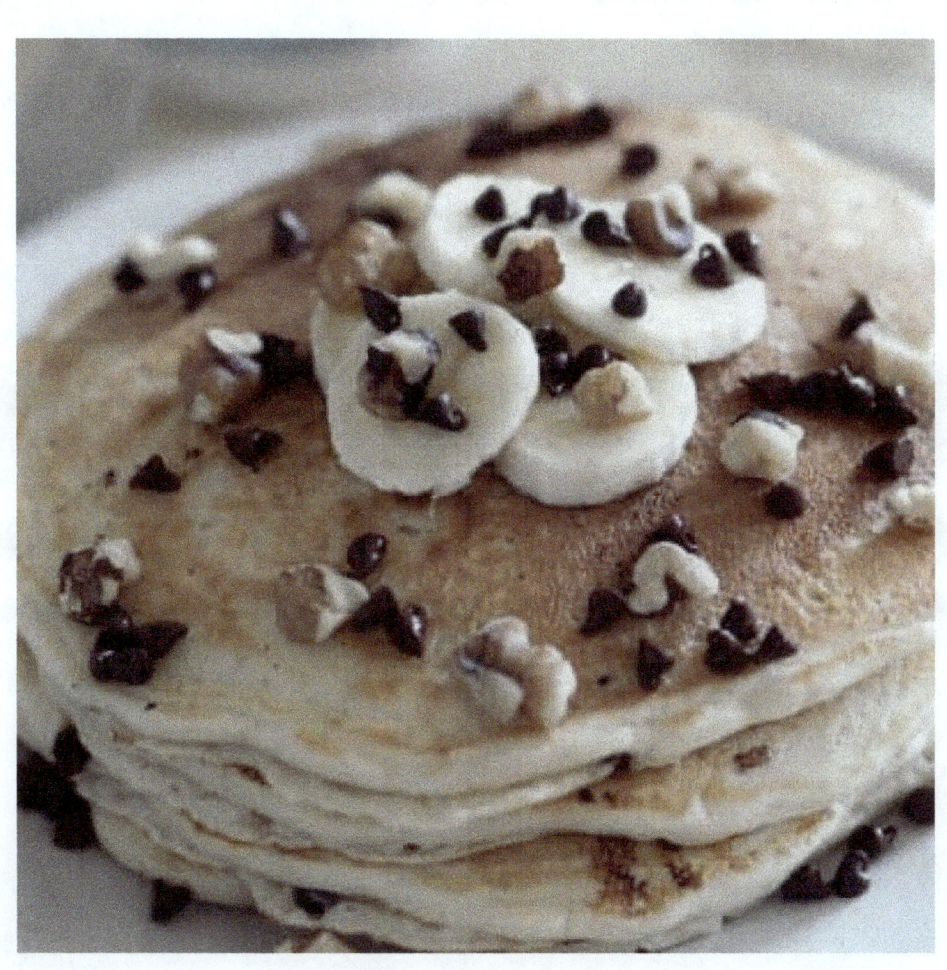

Creamy Oats, Greens and Blueberry Smoothie

Preparation Time: 4 minutes

Cooking Time: 0 minutes

Servings: 1

Ingredients:

- 1 c. cold
- Fat-free milk
- 1 c. salad greens
- 1/2 c. fresh froze. blueberries
- 1/2 c. froze. cooked oatmeal
- 1 tbsp.... sunflower seeds

Directions:

1. Merge all ingredients and blend until smooth and creamy.
2. Serve and enjoy.

Nutrition:

Calories: 280

Fat: 6.8 g

Carbs: 44.0 g

Protein: 14.0 g

Carrot and Bran Mini Muffins

Preparation Time: 10 minutes

Cooking Time: 18 minutes

Servings: 18

Ingredients:

- Nonstick cooking spray
- 1 cup oat bran
- 1 cup whole-wheat flo ur
- 1/2 cup all-purpose flour
- 1/2 cup old-fashioned oats
- 3 tablespoons packed brown sugar
- 1 teaspoon baking soda
- 1 teaspoon baking powder
- 2 teaspoons ground cinnamon
- 2 teaspoons ground ginger
- 1/2 teaspoon ground nutmeg
- 1/4 teaspoon sea salt
- 11/4 cups unsweetened almond milk
- 2 tablespoons honey
- 1 egg
- 2 tablespoons extra-virgin olive oil
- 11/2 cups grated carrots
- 1/4 cup raisins

Directions:

1. Preheat the oven to 350°F.
2. Coat with nonstick cooking spray.
3. In a large bowl, whisk the oat bran, whole-wheat and all-purpose flours, oats, brown sugar, baking soda, baking powder, cinnamon, ginger, nutmeg, and salt. Set aside.
4. Whip the almond milk, honey, egg, and olive oil.
5. Merge all ingredients and fold until just blended. The batter will be lumpy with streaks of flour remaining.
6. Fold in the carrots and raisins.
7. Fill each muffin cup three-fourths full.
8. Cool on a wire rack before serving.

Nutrition:

Calories: 115 ; Protein: 2g ; Total Carbohydrates: 20g ; Fiber: 1g, Total Fat: 3g; Saturated Fat: 1g; Sodium: 178mg

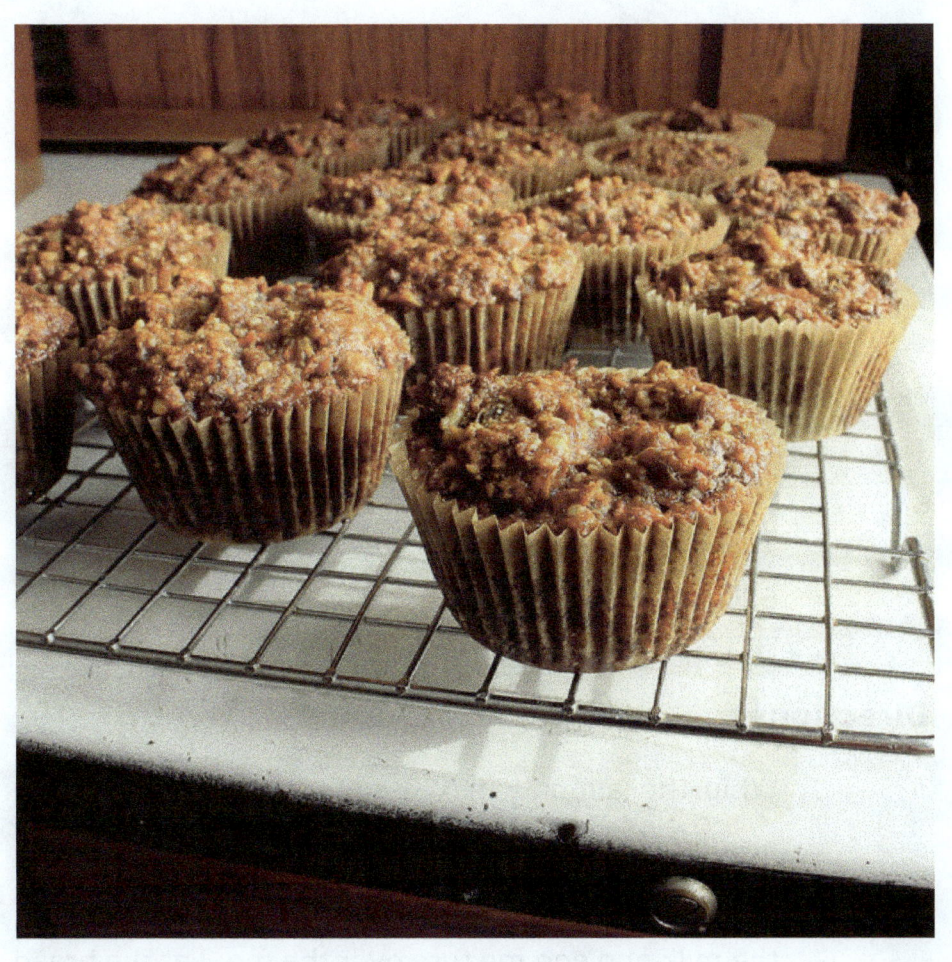

French toast

Preparation Time: 6 minutes

Cooking Time: 20 minutes

Servings: 10

Ingredients:

- 1 1/2 cups unsweetened almond milk
- 2 eggs, beaten
- 2 egg whites, beaten
- 1 teaspoon vanilla extract
- Zest of 1 orange
- Juice of 1 orange
- 1 teaspoon ground nutmeg
- 6 light whole-wheat bread slices
- Nonstick cooking spray

Directions:

1. Whip the almond milk, eggs, egg whites, vanilla, orange zest and juice, and nutmeg.
2. Set the bread in a 9-by-13-inch baking dish. Pour the milk and egg mixture over the top. Let the bread to dip for about 10 minutes, turning once.
3. Drizzle a nonstick skillet with cooking spray and heat over medium-high heat. Working in batches,

add the bread and cook for about 5 minutes per side until the custard sets.

Nutrition:

Calories: 223

Protein: 8g

Total Carbohydrates: 15g

Fiber: 5g

Total Fat: 21g

Saturated Fat: 13g

Sodium: 126mg

Jolene's Green Juice

Preparation Time: 15 minutes

Cooking Time: None

Servings: 3

Ingredients:

- 3 cups dark leafy greens
- 1 cucumber
- 1/4 cup fresh Italian parsley leaves
- 1/4 pineapple, cut into wedges
- 1/2 green apple
- 1/2 orange
- 1/2 lemon

Directions:

1. Pinch grated fresh ginger
2. Using a juicer, run the greens, cucumber, parsley, pineapple, apple, orange, lemon, and ginger through it, pour into a large cup, and serve.

Nutrition:

Calories: 108

Protein: 11g

Total Carbohydrates: 29g

Total Fat: 2g

Sodium: 119mg

Chocolate Banana Smoothie

Preparation Time: 5 minutes

Cooking Time: None

Servings: 3

Ingredients:

- 2 bananas, peeled
- 1 cup unsweetened almond milk
- 1 cup crushed ice
- 3 tablespoons unsweetened cocoa powder
- 3 tablespoons honey

Directions:

1. In a blender, merge the bananas, almond milk, ice, cocoa powder, and honey. Blend until smooth.

Nutrition:

Calories: 219

Protein: 2g

Total Carbohydrates: 57g

Sodium: 4mg

Mediterranean Frittata

Preparation Time: 5 minutes

Cooking Time: 25 minutes

Servings: 2

Ingredients:

- Eggs, six
- Black pepper, one-quarter of a teaspoon
- Milk, one-quarter of a cup
- Oregano, one teaspoon
- Tomatoes, one-quarter of a cup, diced
- Salt, one teaspoon
- Green olives, one-quarter of a cup, chopped finely
- Feta cheese, one-quarter of a cup, crumble
- Black olives, one-quarter of a cup, chopped finely

Directions:

1. Heat the oven to 400. Spray oil an eight-by-eight-inch baking dish. Beat the milk into the eggs, and then add the other ingredients. Pour this mixture into the baking dish and bake for twenty minutes.

Nutrition:

Calories 107

7 grams fat

705 milligrams sodium

3 grams carbs

2 grams sugars

7 grams protein

Mediterranean Eggs

Preparation Time: 5 minutes

Cooking Time: 1 hour and 18 minutes

Servings: 2

Ingredients:

- Yellow onion, one large, cut in thin slices
- Parsley, one-quarter of a cup, chopped finely
- Butter, one tablespoon
- Sea salt, one-quarter of a teaspoon
- Olive oil, one tablespoon
- Black pepper, one-half of a teaspoon
- Garlic, one clove, chopped fine
- Feta cheese, three ounces, crumbled small
- Tomatoes, one-half of a cup, cut in thin slices
- Eggs, eight

Directions:

1. Cook the onions in the butter until they are soft for about ten minutes.
2. Stir in the olive oil, along with the tomatoes and garlic and cook for five more minutes.
3. Lower the heat and break the eggs over the mix, drizzling with pepper, salt, and feta.

4. Cover and cook for ten minutes without stirring over low heat.
5. Sprinkle on the parsley and serve.

Nutrition:

Calories 183, 11 grams carbs, 9 grams protein, 11 grams fat, 255 milligrams sodium, 1 gram fiber, 6 grams sugar

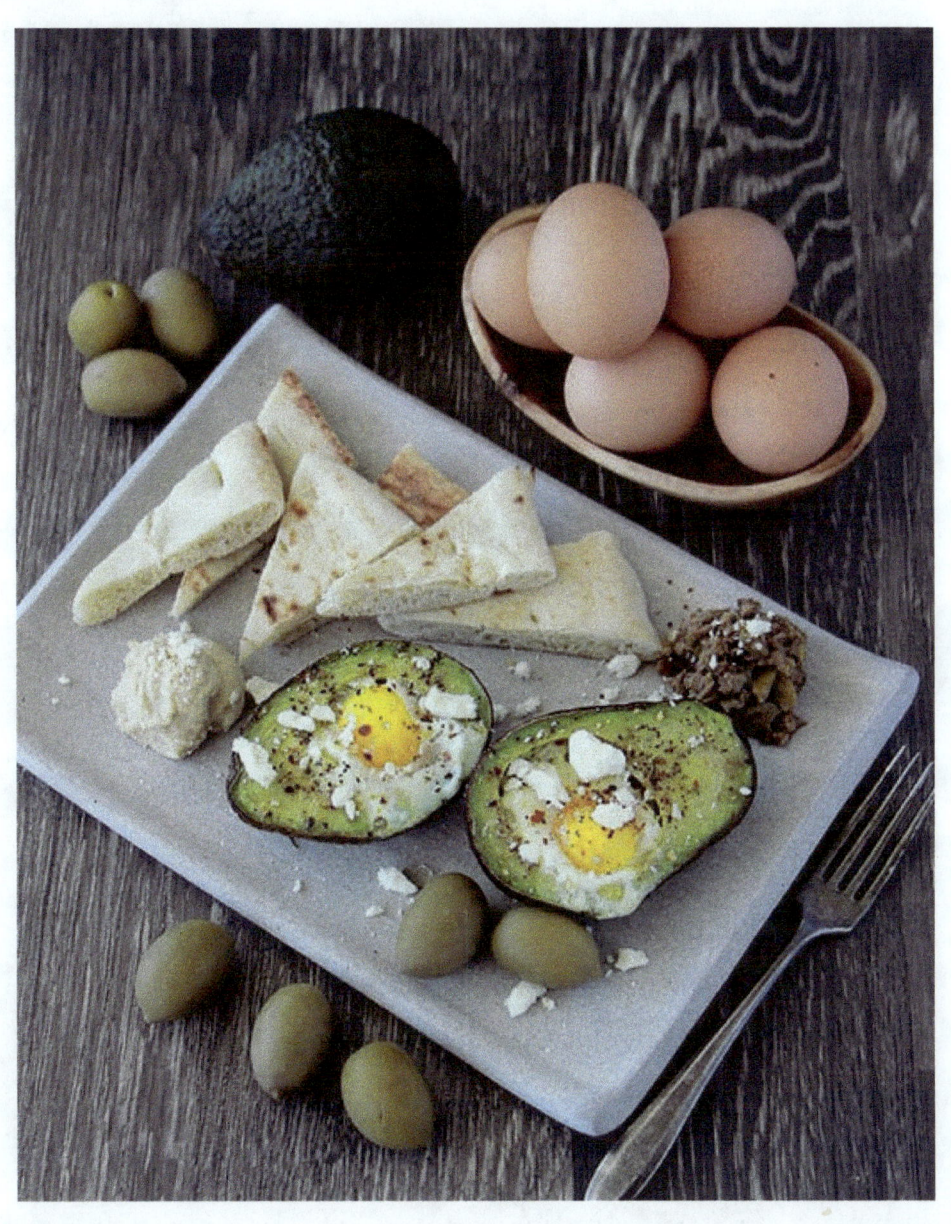

Southwest Tofu Scramble

Preparation Time: 10 minutes

Cooking Time: 20 minutes

Servings: 2

Ingredients:

- Kale, two cups, washed, dried, and chopped into small pieces
- Eggs, four, beaten well
- Red pepper, one-half of one, sliced thinly
- Olive oil, two tablespoons
- Red onion, one-fourth of one, sliced thinly
- Garlic powder, one teaspoon
- Turmeric, a quarter teaspoon
- Water, just enough to thin ingredients
- Chili powder, a quarter teaspoon
- Sea salt, one-half teaspoon
- Cumin powder, one-half teaspoon

Directions:

1. To make the sauce, mix all of the spices together in a bowl, and add just enough water to stir into a sauce-type of consistency.
2. Cook the red pepper, kale, and onion for three to four minutes in the olive oil.

3. Then pour the beaten egg all over the mix in the pan, and cook it until the eggs reach your desired set.

Nutrition:

Calories 252

19 grams fat

516 milligrams sodium

12.7 grams carbs

3 grams fiber

2.5 grams sugar

12 grams protein

Mediterranean Breakfast Salad

Preparation Time: 30 minutes

Cooking Time: 0 minutes

Servings: 2

Ingredients:

- Eggs, four, hard-boiled and sliced in thin slices
- Lemon juice, three tablespoons
- Arugula, ten cups, washed and d ried
- Olive oil, two tablespoons
- Tomato, one large, cut into eight wedges
- Dill, one-half of a cup, chopped finely
- Cucumber, one-half of a cup, chopped finely
- Almonds, one cup, chopped finely
- Quinoa, one cup, cooked and already cooled
- Avocado, one large, sliced in thin slices

Directions:

1. Mix the quinoa with the tomatoes, cucumber, and arugula.
2. Add the salt, pepper, and olive oil; toss lightly.
3. Place the salad mix on four salad plates, arrange the sliced egg and the avocado slices on top of the salad mix, and top with the almonds and herbs.
4. Drizzle the lemon juice all over it.

Nutrition:

Calories 336, 7.7 grams fat, 946.4 milligrams sodium, 54.6 grams carbs, 5.2 grams fiber, 5.5 grams sugar, 12.3 grams protein

Lunch

Easy Tuna Patties

Preparation Time: 15 minutes

Cooking Time: 10 minutes

Servings: 2

Ingredients:

- 2 teaspoons lemon juice
- 3 tablespoons grated Parmesan
- 2 eggs
- 10 tablespoons Italian breadcrumbs
- 3 tuna cans, drained
- 3 tablespoons diced onion
- 1 pinch of ground black pepper
- 3 tablespoons vegetable oil

Directions:

1. Beat the eggs and lemon juice in a bowl. Stir in the Parmesan cheese and breadcrumbs to obtain a paste. Add tuna and onion until everything is well mixed. Season with black pepper. Form the tuna mixture into eight 1-inch-thick patties.
2. Heat the vegetable oil in a frying pan over medium heat; fry the patties until golden brown, about 5 minutes on each side.

Nutrition:

325 calories

15.5 grams of fat

13.9 g of carbohydrates

31.3 g of protein

125 mg cholesterol

409 mg of sodium

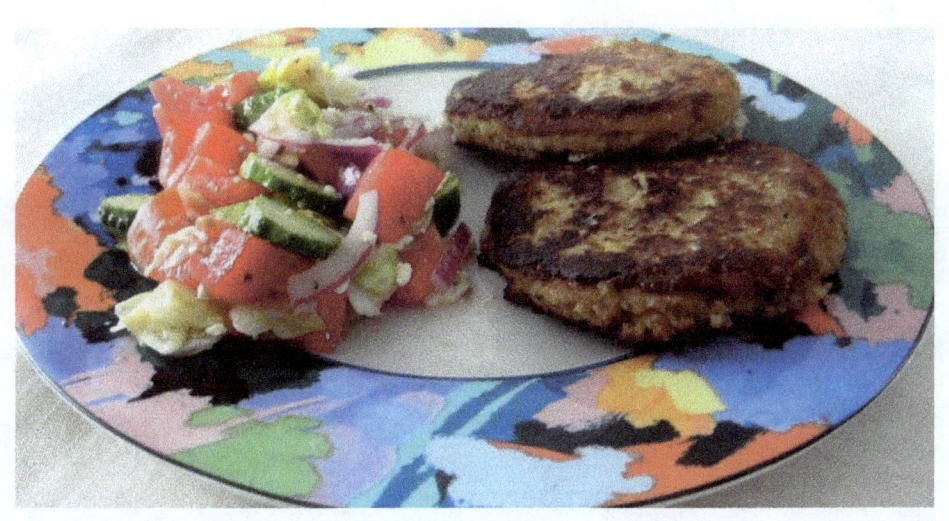

Fish Tacos

Preparation Time: 40 minutes

Cooking Time: 15 minutes

Servings: 2

Ingredients:

- 1 cup flour
- 2 tablespoons corn flour
- 1 teaspoon baking powder
- 1/2 teaspoon of salt
- 1 egg
- 1 cup of beer
- 1/2 cup of yogurt
- 1/2 cup of mayonnaise
- 1 lime, juice
- 1 jalapeño pepper, minced
- 1 c. Finely chopped capers
- 1/2 teaspoon dried oregano
- 1/2 teaspoon ground cumin
- 1/2 teaspoon dried dill
- 1 teaspoon ground cayenne pepper
- 1 liter of oil for frying
- 1 pound of cod fillets, 2-3 ounces each
- 8 corn tortillas

- 1/2 medium cabbage, finely shredded

Directions:

1. Prepare beer dough: combine flour, corn flour, baking powder and salt in a large bowl. Mix the egg and the beer and stir in the flour mixture quickly.
2. To make a white sauce: combine yogurt and mayonnaise in a medium bowl. Gradually add fresh lime juice until it is slightly fluid — season with jalapeño, capers, oregano, cumin, dill, and cayenne pepper.
3. Heat the oil in a frying pan.
4. Lightly sprinkle the fish with flour. Dip it in the beer batter and fry until crispy and golden brown. Drain on kitchen paper. Heat the tortillas. Place the fried fish in a tortilla and garnish with grated cabbage and white sauce.

Nutrition:

409 calories; 18.8 g of fat; 43 grams of carbohydrates ; 17.3 g of protein; 54 mg cholesterol; 407 mg of sodium

Blackened Salmon Fillets

Preparation Time: 15 minutes
Cooking Time: 10 minutes
Servings: 2

Ingredients:

- 2 tablespoons paprika powder
- 1 tablespoon cayenne pepper powder
- 1 tablespoon onion powder
- 2 teaspoons salt
- 1/2 teaspoon ground white pepper
- 1/2 teaspoon ground black pepper
- 1/4 teaspoon dried thyme
- 1/4 teaspoon dried basil
- 1/4 teaspoon dried oregano
- 4 salmon fillets, skin and bones removed
- 1/2 cup unsalted butter, melted

Directions:

1. Combine bell pepper, cayenne pepper, onion powder, salt, white pepper, black pepper, thyme, basil and oregano in a small bowl.
2. Brush salmon fillets with 1/4 cup butter and sprinkle evenly with the cayenne pepper mixture. Sprinkle each fillet with ½ of the remaining butter.

3. Cook the salmon in a large heavy-bottomed pan, until dark, 2 to 5 minutes. Turn the fillets, sprinkle with the remaining butter and continue to cook until the fish easily peels with a fork.

Nutrition:

511 calories

38.3 grams of fat

4.5 grams of carbohydrates

37.4 g of protein

166 mg cholesterol

1248 mg of sodium

Brown Butter Perch

Preparation Time: 15 minutes

Cooking Time: 10 minutes

Servings: 2

Ingredients:

- 1 cup flour
- 1 teaspoon salt
- 1/2 teaspoon finely ground black pepper
- 1/2 teaspoon cayenne pepper
- 8 oz. fresh perch fillets
- 2 tablespoons butter
- 1 lemon cut in half

Directions:

1. In a bowl, beat flour, salt, black pepper, and cayenne pepper. Gently squeeze the perch fillets into the flour mixture to coat well and remove excess flour.
2. Heat the butter in a frying pan over medium heat until it is foamy and brown hazel. Place the fillets in portions in the pan and cook them light brown, about 2 minutes on each side. Place the cooked fillets on a plate, squeeze the lemon juice, and serve.

Nutrition:

271 calories

11.5 g of fat

30.9 g of carbohydrates

12.6 g of protein

43 mg of cholesterol

703 mg of sodium

Almond Crust Chicken

Preparation Time: 10 minutes

Cooking Time: 25 minutes

Servings: 2

Ingredients:

- 2 chicken breasts, skinless and boneless
- 1 tbsp Dijon mustard
- 2 tbsp mayonnaise
- ¼ cup almonds
- Pepper
- Salt

Directions:

1. Add almond into the food processor and process until finely ground.
2. Transfer almonds on a plate and set aside.
3. Mix together mustard and mayonnaise and spread over chicken.
4. Coat chicken with almond and place into the air fryer basket and cook at 350 F for 25 minutes.
5. Serve and enjoy.

Nutrition:

Calories 409

Fat 22 g

Carbohydrates 6 g

Sugar 1.5 g

Protein 45 g

Cholesterol 134 mg

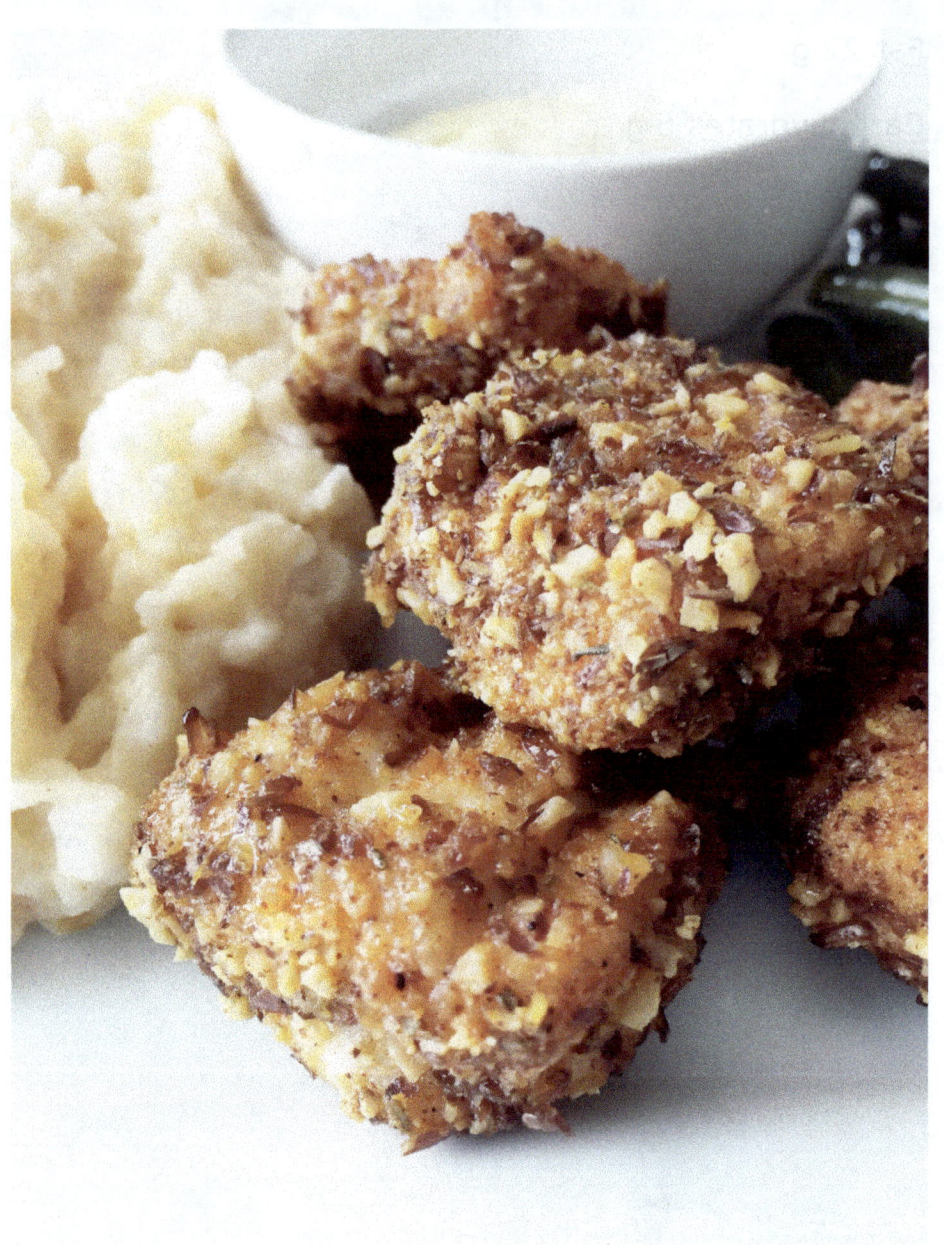

Mushroom Cheese Salad

Preparation Time: 10 minutes

Cooking Time: 15 minutes

Servings: 2

Ingredients:

- 10 mushrooms, halved
- 1 tbsp. fresh parsley, chopped
- 1 tbsp. olive oil
- 1 tbsp. mozzarella cheese, grated
- 1 tbsp. cheddar cheese, grated
- 1 tbsp. dried mix herbs
- Pepper
- Salt

Directions:

1. Add all Ingredients into the bowl and toss well.
2. Transfer bowl mixture into the air fryer baking dish.
3. Place in the air fryer and cook at 380 F for 15 minutes.
4. Serve and enjoy.

Nutrition:

Calories: 90

Fat: 7 g

Carbohydrates: 2 g

Sugar: 1 g

Protein: 5 g

Cholesterol: 7 mg

Shrimp Sandwiches

Preparation Time: 10 minutes

Cooking Time: 5 minutes

Servings: 2

Ingredients:

- 1 and ¼ cups cheddar, shredded
- 6 ounces canned tiny shrimp, drained
- 3 tablespoons mayonnaise
- 2 tablespoons green onions, chopped
- 4 whole wheat bread slices
- 2 tablespoons butter, soft

Directions:

1. In a bowl, mix shrimp with cheese, green onion and mayo and stir well. Spread this on half of the bread slices, top with the other bread slices, cut into halves diagonally and spread butter on top. Place sandwiches in your air fryer and cook at 350 degrees F for 5 minutes. Divide shrimp sandwiches on plates and serve them for breakfast. Enjoy!

Nutrition:

Calories: 162

Fat: 3

Fiber: 7

Carbs: 12

Protein: 4

Asparagus Salad

Preparation Time: 5 minutes

Cooking Time: 10 minutes

Servings: 4

Ingredients:

- 1 cup baby arugula
- 1 bunch asparagus; trimmed
- 1 tbsp. balsamic vinegar
- 1 tbsp. cheddar cheese; grated
- A pinch of salt and black pepper
- Cooking spray

Directions:

1. Put the asparagus in your air fryer's basket, grease with cooking spray, season with salt and pepper and cook at 360°F for 10 minutes.
2. Take a bowl and mix the asparagus with the arugula and the vinegar, toss, divide between plates and serve hot with cheese sprinkled on top

Nutrition:

Calories: 200

Fat: 5g

Fiber: 1g

Carbs: 4g

Protein: 5g

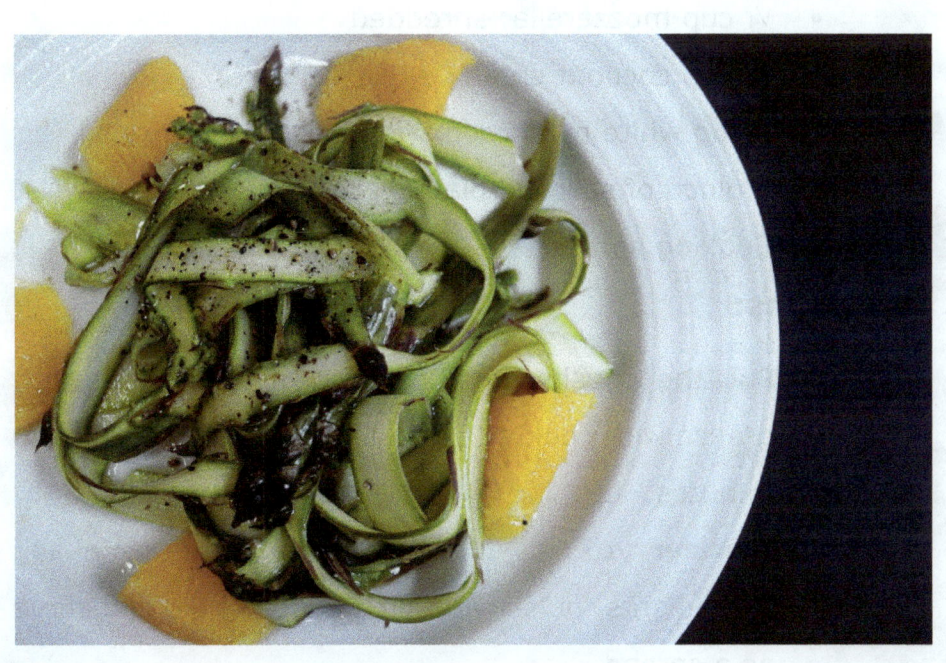

Mushrooms and Cheese Spread

Preparation Time: 5 minutes

Cooking Time: 20 minutes

Servings: 4

Ingredients:

- ¼ cup mozzarella; shredded
- ½ cup coconut cream
- 1 cup white mushrooms
- A pinch of salt and black pepper
- Cooking spray

Directions:

1. Put the mushrooms in your air fryer's basket, grease with cooking spray and cook at 370°F for 20 minutes.
2. Transfer to a blender, add the remaining Ingredients, pulse well, divide into bowls and serve as a spread

Nutrition:

Calories: 202

Fat: 12g

Fiber: 2g

Carbs: 5g

Protein: 7g

Italian Baked Beans

Preparation Time: 5 minutes

Cooking Time: 15 minutes

Servings: 6

Ingredients:

- 2 teaspoons extra-virgin olive oil
- ½ cup minced onion (about ¼ onion)
- 1 (12-ounce) can low-sodium tomato paste
- ¼ cup red wine vinegar
- 2 tablespoons honey
- ¼ teaspoon ground cinnamon
- ½ cup water
- 2 (15-ounce) cans cannellini or great northern beans, undrained

Directions:

1. In a medium saucepan over medium heat, heat the oil. Add the onion and cook for 5 minutes, stirring frequently.
2. Add the tomato paste, vinegar, honey, cinnamon, and water, and mix well. Turn the heat to low. Drain and rinse one can of the beans in a colander and add to the saucepan.

3. Pour the entire second can of beans (including the liquid) into the saucepan. Let it cook for 10 minutes, stirring occasionally, and serve.
4. Ingredient tip: Switch up this recipe by making new variations of the homemade ketchup. Instead of the cinnamon, try ¼ teaspoon of smoked paprika and 1 tablespoon of hot sauce. Serve.

Nutrition:

Calories: 236

Fat: 3g

Carbohydrates: 42g

Protein: 10g

Cannellini Bean Lettuce Wraps

Preparation Time: 15 minutes

Cooking Time: 10 minutes

Servings: 4

Ingredients:

- 1 tablespoon extra-virgin olive oil
- ½ cup diced red onion (about ¼ onion)
- ¾ cup chopped fresh tomatoes (about 1 medium tomato)
- ¼ teaspoon freshly ground black pepper
- 1 (15-ounce) can cannellini or great northern beans, drained and rinsed
- ¼ cup finely chopped fresh curly parsley
- ½ cup Lemony Garlic Hummus or ½ cup prepared hummus
- 8 romaine lettuce leaves

Directions:

1. In a large skillet over medium heat, heat the oil. Add the onion and cook for 3 minutes, stirring occasionally.
2. Add the tomatoes and pepper and cook for 3 more minutes, stirring occasionally. Add the beans and

cook for 3 more minutes, stirring occasionally. Remove from the heat, and mix in the parsley.
3. Spread 1 tablespoon of hummus over each lettuce leaf. Evenly spread the warm bean mixture down the center of each leaf.
4. Fold one side of the lettuce leaf over the filling lengthwise, then fold over the other side to make a wrap and serve.

Nutrition:

Calories: 211

Fat: 8g

Carbohydrates: 28g

Protein: 10g

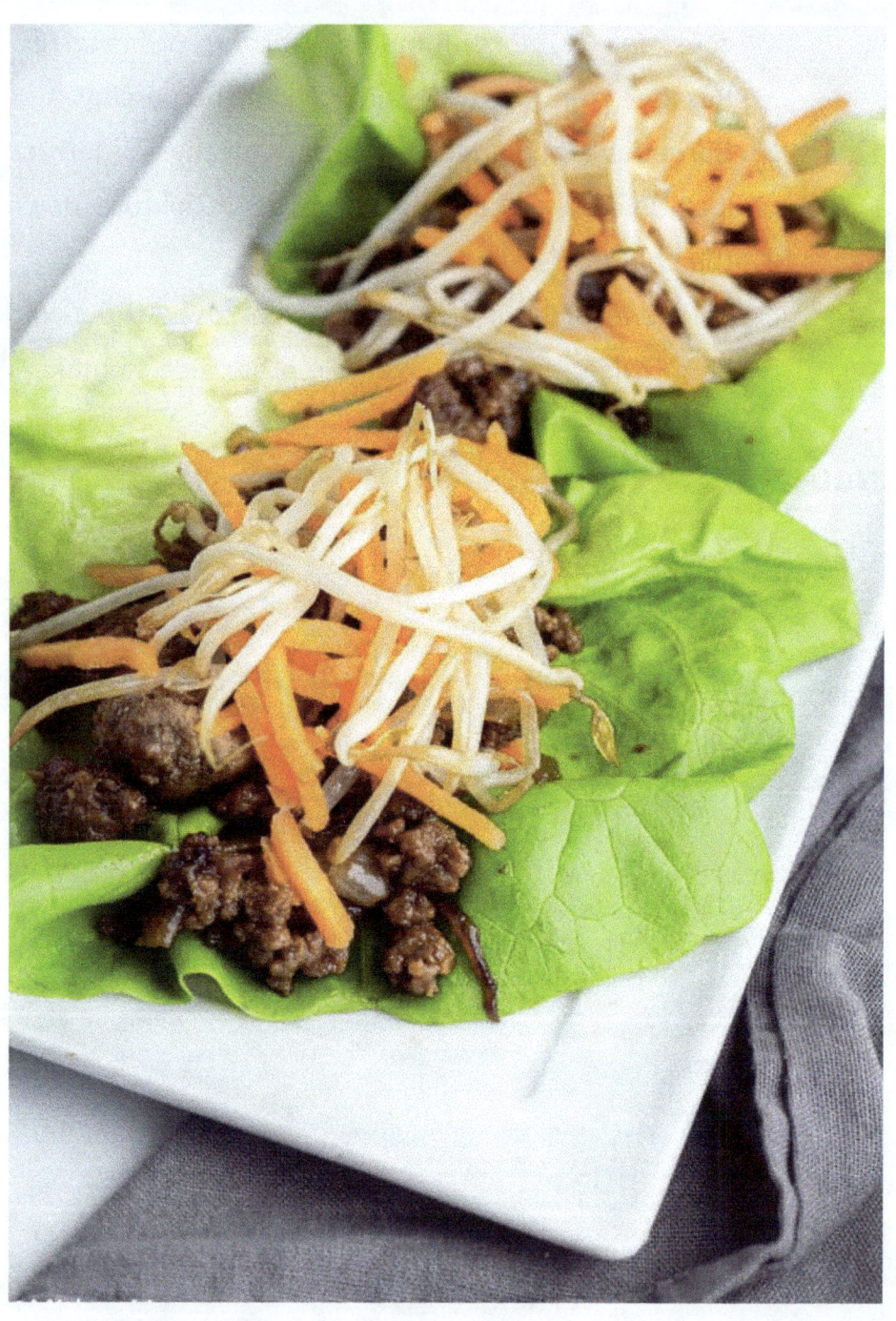

Israeli Eggplant, Chickpea, and Mint Sauté

Preparation Time: 5 minutes

Cooking Time: 20 minutes

Servings: 6

Ingredients:

- Nonstick cooking spray
- 1 medium globe eggplant (about 1 pound), stem removed
- 1 tablespoon extra-virgin olive oil
- 2 tablespoons freshly squeezed lemon juice (from about 1 small lemon)
- 2 tablespoons balsamic vinegar
- 1 teaspoon ground cumin
- ¼ teaspoon kosher or sea salt
- 1 (15-ounce) can chickpeas, drained and rinsed
- 1 cup sliced sweet onion (about ½ medium Walla Walla or Vidalia onion)
- ¼ cup loosely packed chopped or torn mint leaves
- 1 tablespoon sesame seeds, toasted if desired
- 1 garlic clove, finely minced (about ½ teaspoon)

Directions:

1. Place one oven rack about 4 inches below the broiler element. Turn the broiler to the highest setting to preheat. Spray a large, rimmed baking sheet with nonstick cooking spray.
2. On a cutting board, cut the eggplant lengthwise into four slabs (each piece should be about ½- to 1/8-inch thick). Place the eggplant slabs on the prepared baking sheet. Set aside.
3. In a small bowl, whisk together the oil, lemon juice, vinegar, cumin, and salt. Brush or drizzle 2 tablespoons of the lemon dressing over both sides of the eggplant slabs. Reserve the remaining dressing.
4. Broil the eggplant directly under the heating element for 4 minutes, flip them, then broil for another 4 minutes, until golden brown.
5. While the eggplant is broiling, in a serving bowl, combine the chickpeas, onion, mint, sesame seeds, and garlic. Add the reserved dressing, and gently mix to incorporate all the ingredients.
6. When the eggplant is done, using tongs, transfer the slabs from the baking sheet to a cooling rack and cool for 3 minutes.

7. When slightly cooled, place the eggplant on a cutting board and slice each slab crosswise into ½-inch strips.
8. Add the eggplant to the serving bowl with the onion mixture. Gently toss everything together, and serve warm or at room temperature.

Nutrition:

Calories: 159

Fat: 4g

Carbohydrates: 26g

Protein: 6g

Minestrone Chickpeas and Macaroni Casserole

Preparation Time: 15 minutes

Cooking Time: 7 hours & 25 minutes

Servings: 5

Ingredients:

- 1 (15-ounce / 425-g) can chickpeas, drained and rinsed
- 1 (28-ounce / 794-g) can diced tomatoes, with the juice
- 1 (6-ounce / 170-g) can no-salt-added tomato paste
- 3 medium carrots, sliced
- 3 cloves garlic, minced
- 1 medium yellow onion, chopped
- 1 cup low-sodium vegetable soup
- ½ teaspoon dried rosemary
- 1 teaspoon dried oregano
- 2 teaspoons maple syrup
- ½ teaspoon sea salt
- ¼ teaspoon ground black pepper

- ½ pound (227-g) fresh green beans, trimmed and cut into bite-size pieces
- 1 cup macaroni pasta
- 2 ounces (57 g) Parmesan cheese, grated

Directions:

1. Except for the green beans, pasta, and Parmesan cheese, combine all the ingredients in the slow cooker and stir to mix well. Put the slow cooker lid on and cook on low for 7 hours.
2. Fold in the pasta and green beans. Put the lid on and cook on high for 20 minutes or until the vegetable are soft and the pasta is al dente.
3. Pour them in a large serving bowl and spread with Parmesan cheese before serving.

Nutrition:

Calories: 349, Fat: 6.7g, Protein: 16.5g, Carbs: 59.9g

Mediterranean Lentils and Rice

Preparation Time: 5 minutes

Cooking Time: 25 minutes

Servings: 4

Ingredients:

- 2¼ cups low-sodium or no-salt-added vegetable broth
- ½ cup uncooked brown or green lentils
- ½ cup uncooked instant brown rice
- ½ cup diced carrots (about 1 carrot)
- ½ cup diced celery (about 1 stalk)
- 1 (2.25-ounce) can sliced olives, drained (about ½ cup)
- ¼ cup diced red onion (about 1/8 onion)
- ¼ cup chopped fresh curly-leaf parsley
- 1½ tablespoons extra-virgin olive oil
- 1 tablespoon freshly squeezed lemon juice (from about ½ small lemon)
- 1 garlic clove, minced (about ½ teaspoon)
- ¼ teaspoon kosher or sea salt
- ¼ teaspoon freshly ground black pepper

Directions:

1. In a medium saucepan over high heat, bring the broth and lentils to a boil, cover, and lower the heat to medium-low. Cook for 8 minutes.
2. Raise the heat to medium, and stir in the rice. Cover the pot and cook the mixture for 15 minutes, or until the liquid is absorbed. Remove the pot from the heat and let it sit, covered, for 1 minute, then stir. While the lentils and rice are cooking, mix together the carrots, celery, olives, onion, and parsley in a large serving bowl.
3. In a small bowl, whisk together the oil, lemon juice, garlic, salt, and pepper. Set aside. When the lentils and rice are cooked, add them to the serving bowl.
4. Pour the dressing on top, and mix everything together. Serve warm or cold, or store in a sealed container in the refrigerator for up to 7 days.

Nutrition:

Calories: 230; Fat: 8g; Carbohydrates: 34g; Protein: 8g

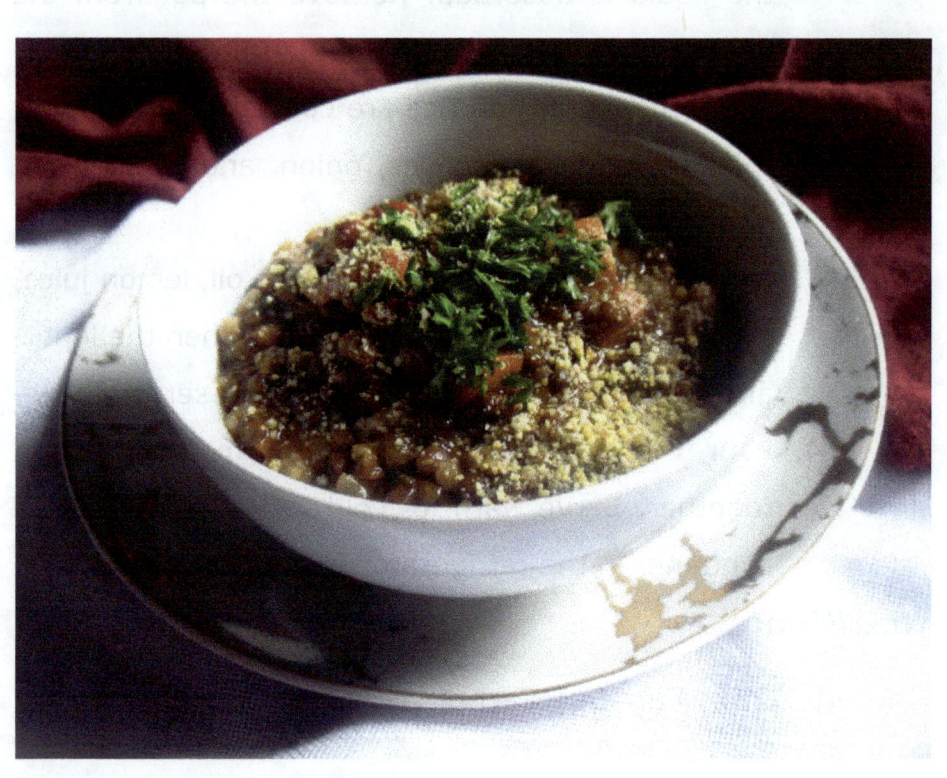

Polenta with Sautéed Chard and Fried Eggs

Preparation Time: 5 minutes

Cooking Time: 20 minutes

Servings: 4

Ingredients:

- 2½ cups water
- ½ teaspoon kosher salt
- ¾ cups whole-grain cornmeal
- ¼ teaspoon freshly ground black pepper
- 2 tablespoons grated Parmesan cheese
- 1 tablespoon extra-virgin olive oil
- 1 bunch (about 6 ounces) Swiss chard, leaves and stems chopped and separated
- 2 garlic cloves, sliced
- ¼ teaspoon kosher salt
- 1/8 teaspoon freshly ground black pepper
- Lemon juice (optional)
- 1 tablespoon extra-virgin olive oil
- 4 large eggs

Directions:

1. For the polenta, bring the water and salt to a boil in a medium saucepan over high heat. Slowly add the cornmeal, whisking constantly.
2. Decrease the heat to low, cover, and cook for 10 to 15 minutes, stirring often to avoid lumps. Stir in the pepper and Parmesan and divide among 4 bowls.
3. For the chard, heat the oil in a large skillet over medium heat. Add the chard stems, garlic, salt, and pepper; sauté for 2 minutes. Add the chard leaves and cook until wilted, about 3 to 5 minutes.
4. Add a spritz of lemon juice (if desired), toss together, and divide evenly on top of the polenta.
5. For the eggs, heat the oil in the same large skillet over medium-high heat. Crack each egg into the skillet, taking care not to crowd the skillet and leaving space between the eggs.
6. Cook until the whites are set and golden around the edges, about 2 to 3 minutes. Serve sunny-side up or flip the eggs over carefully and cook 1 minute longer for over easy. Place one egg on top of the polenta and chard in each bowl.

Nutrition:

Calories: 310; Protein: 17 g; Fat: 18 g; Carbs: 21 g

Dinner

Simple Beef Sirloin Roast

Preparation Time: 10 minutes

Cooking Time: 50 minutes

Servings: 8

Ingredients:

- 2½ pounds sirloin roast
- Salt and ground black pepper, as required

Directions:

1. Rub the roast with salt and black pepper generously.
2. Insert the rotisserie rod through the roast.
3. Insert the rotisserie forks, one on each side of the rod to secure the rod to the chicken.
4. Arrange the drip pan in the bottom of Air Fryer Oven cooking chamber.
5. Select "Roast" and then adjust the temperature to 350 degrees F.
6. Set the timer for 50 minutes and press the "Start".
7. When the display shows "Add Food" press the red lever down and load the left side of the rod into the Air fryer oven.
8. Now, slide the rod's left side into the groove along the metal bar so it doesn't move. Then, close the

door and touch "Rotate". Press the red lever to release the rod when cooking time is complete.
9. Remove from the Air fryer oven and place the roast onto a platter for about 10 minutes before slicing. With a sharp knife, cut the roast into desired sized slices and serve.

Nutrition:

Calories 201

Fat 8.8 g

Carbs 0 g

Protein 28.9 g

Garlicky Pork Tenderloin

Preparation Time: 15 minutes

Cooking Time: 20 minutes

Servings: 5

Ingredients:

- 1½ pounds pork tenderloin
- Nonstick cooking spray
- 2 small heads roasted garlic
- Salt and ground black pepper, as required

Directions:

1. Lightly, spray all the sides of pork with cooking spray and then, season with salt and black pepper.
2. Now, rub the pork with roasted garlic. Arrange the roast onto the lightly greased cooking tray.
3. Arrange the drip pan in the bottom of Air Fryer Oven cooking chamber.
4. Select "Air Fry" and then adjust the temperature to 400 degrees F. Set the timer for 20 minutes and press the "Start".
5. When the display shows "Add Food" insert the cooking tray in the center position.
6. When the display shows "Turn Food" turn the pork.

7. When cooking time is complete, remove the tray from Air fryer oven and place the roast onto a platter for about 10 minutes before slicing. With a sharp knife, cut the roast into desired sized slices and serve.

Nutrition:

Calories 202

Fat 4.8 g

Carbs 1.7 g

Protein 35.9 g

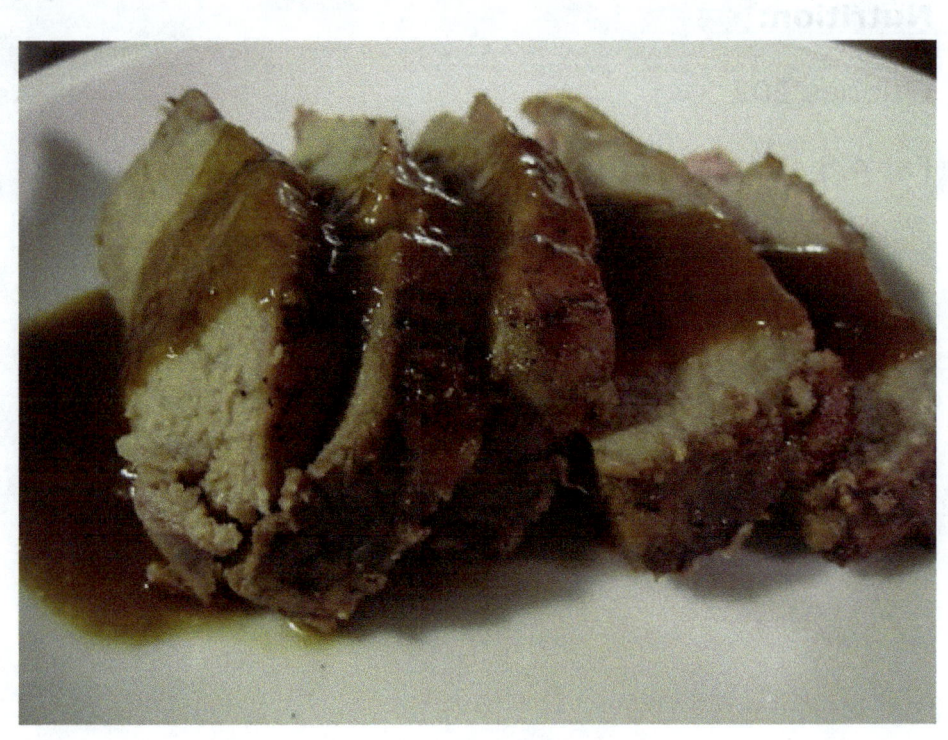

Greek Lamb Chops

Preparation Time: 10 minutes

Cooking Time: 10 minutes

Servings: 4

Ingredients:

- 2 lbs. lamb chops
- 2 tsp garlic, minced
- 1 ½ tsp dried oregano
- ¼ cup fresh lemon juice
- ¼ cup olive oil
- ½ tsp pepper
- 1 tsp salt

Directions:

1. Add lamb chops in a mixing bowl. Add remaining ingredients over the lamb chops and coat well.
2. Arrange lamb chops on the air fryer oven tray and cook at 400 F for 5 minutes
3. Turn lamb chops and cook for 5 minutes more.
4. Serve and enjoy.

Nutrition:

Calories 538; Fat 29.4 g; Carbs 1.3 g; Protein 64 g

Delicious Cauliflower Rice

Preparation Time: 10 minutes
Cooking Time: 15 minutes
Servings: 4

Ingredients:

- 10 oz cauliflower rice
- 3 tbsp sun-dried tomatoes, minced
- 2 cups spinach, chopped
- 1/3 cup vegetable broth
- 2 tomatoes, diced
- 1 small zucchini, sliced
- 1 garlic clove, minced
- 1 cup mushrooms, sliced
- ½ small onion, diced
- 2 tbsp olive oil
- Pepper
- Salt

Directions:

1. Heat oil in a pan over medium heat. Add mushrooms and onion and sauté for 5 minutes. Add garlic and sauté for a minute.

2. Add cauliflower rice, tomato, zucchini, and broth and stir well. Cover and cook for 5 minutes or until all liquid evaporates.
3. Add sun-dried tomatoes and spinach and cook for 3-4 minutes. Season with pepper and salt. Serve and enjoy.

Nutrition:

Calories: 107

Fat: 7.5g

Protein: 3.8g

Carbs: 9.1g

Grilled Eggplant

Preparation Time: 10 minutes
Cooking Time: 10 minutes
Servings: 4

Ingredients:

- 2 large eggplants, sliced ¼-inch thick
- ½ lemon juice
- 2 tbsp fresh parsley, chopped
- ¼ cup feta cheese, crumbled
- ¼ tsp chili flakes
- 1 tsp dried oregano
- ½ cup olive oil
- Pepper
- Salt

Directions:

1. Heat grill pan over medium-high heat. In a small bowl, mix together oil, chili flakes, and oregano. Brush eggplants with oil mixture and season with pepper and salt.
2. Place eggplant slices in a grill pan and cook for 3 minutes per side. Transfer grill eggplant slices on serving dish. Drizzle with lemon juice. Top with feta cheese and parsley. Serve and enjoy.

Nutrition:

Calories: 313

Fat: 27.8g

Protein: 4.2g

Carbs: 17g

Flavorful Roasted Vegetables

Preparation Time: 10 minutes
Cooking Time: 30 minutes
Servings: 6

Ingredients:

- 1 eggplant, sliced
- 5 fresh basil leaves, sliced
- 2 tsp Italian seasoning
- 2 tbsp olive oil
- 1 onion, sliced
- 1 bell pepper, cut into strips
- 2 zucchinis, sliced
- 2 tomatoes, quartered
- Pepper
- Salt

Directions:

1. Preheat the oven to 400 F/ 200 C. Line baking tray with parchment paper. Add all ingredients except basil leaves into the mixing bowl and toss well.
2. Transfer veggie mixture on a prepared baking tray and roast in preheated oven for 30 minutes. Garnish with basil leaves and serve.

Nutrition:

Calories: 95

Fat: 5.5g

Protein: 2.3g

Carbs: 11.7g

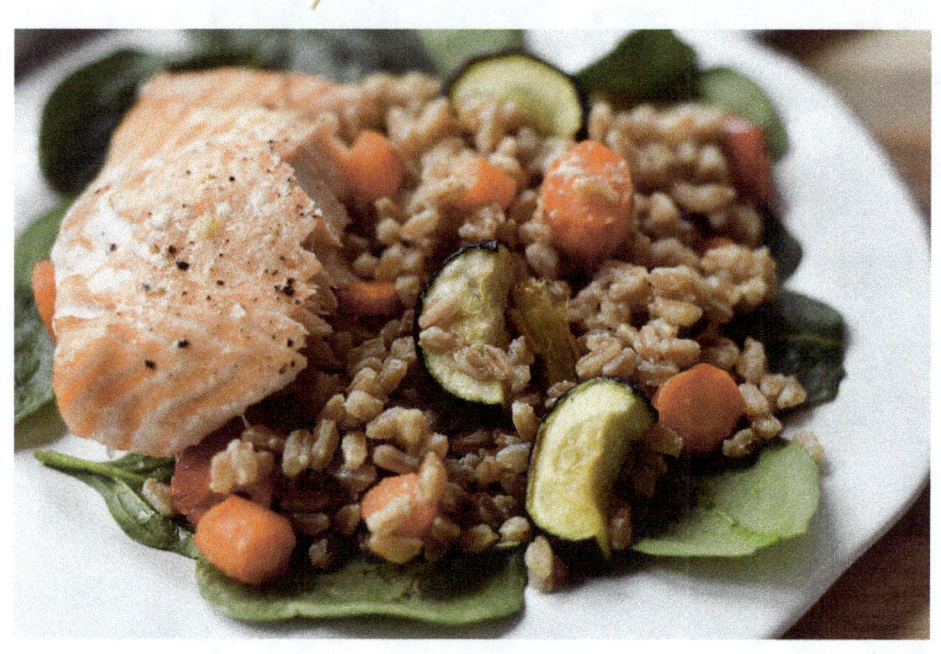

Healthy Carrot Salad

Preparation Time: 10 minutes

Cooking Time: 5 minutes

Servings: 4

Ingredients:

- 1 lb. carrots, peeled and grated
- 1 tsp garlic, minced
- 1 tbsp lemon zest
- ¼ cup fresh lemon juice
- 2 tbsp olive oil
- ¼ tsp cinnamon
- 1 tsp cumin
- 1 tsp sweet paprika
- ¼ cup fresh cilantro, chopped
- ¼ cup fresh parsley, chopped
- ½ cup fresh mint, chopped
- Pepper
- Salt

Directions:

1. Add all ingredients into the mixing bowl and mix until well combined. Serve and enjoy.

Nutrition:

Calories: 123

Fat: 7.4g

Protein: 1.8g

Carbs: 13.9g

Beetroot & Carrot Salad

Preparation Time: 10 minutes

Cooking Time: 5 minutes

Servings: 4

Ingredients:

- 12 oz beetroot, peeled, trimmed, & grated
- 12 oz carrots, peeled, trimmed, & grated
- ¼ cup fresh parsley, chopped
- 1 tbsp red wine vinegar
- 2 tbsp olive oil
- 2 tsp cumin seeds
- 2 shallots, chopped

Directions:

1. Heat oil in a pan over medium heat. Once the oil is hot then add cumin seeds and cook for 30 seconds.
2. Remove pan from heat. Add remaining ingredients to the pan and mix well. Serve and enjoy.

Nutrition:

Calories: 138

Fat: 7.4g

Dill Chutney Salmon

Preparation Time: 5 minutes

Cooking Time: 3 minutes

Servings: 2

Ingredients:

Chutney:

- ¼ cup fresh dill
- ¼ cup extra virgin olive oil
- Juice from ½ lemon
- Sea salt, to taste

Fish:

- 2 cups water
- 2 salmon fillets
- Juice from ½ lemon
- ¼ teaspoon paprika
- Salt and freshly ground pepper to taste

Directions:

1. Pulse all the chutney ingredients in a food processor until creamy. Set aside.
2. Add the water and steamer basket to the Pressure Pot. Place salmon fillets, skin-side down, on the

steamer basket. Drizzle the lemon juice over salmon and sprinkle with the paprika.
3. Secure the lid. Select the Manual mode and set the cooking time for 3 minutes at High Pressure.
4. Once cooking is complete, do a quick pressure release. Carefully open the lid.
5. Season the fillets with pepper and salt to taste. Serve topped with the dill chutney.

Nutrition:

Calories 636,

41g fat,

65g protein

Garlic-Butter Parmesan Salmon and Asparagus

Preparation Time: 10 minutes
Cooking Time: 15 minutes
Servings: 2

Ingredients:

- 2 (6-ounce / 170-g) salmon fillets, skin on and patted dry
- Pink Himalayan salt
- Freshly ground black pepper, to taste
- 1 pound (454 g) fresh asparagus, ends snapped off
- 3 tablespoons almond butter
- 2 garlic cloves, minced
- ¼ cup grated Parmesan cheese

Directions:

1. Prep oven to 400ºF (205ºC). Line a baking sheet with aluminum foil.
2. Season both sides of the salmon fillets.
3. Situate salmon in the middle of the baking sheet and arrange the asparagus around the salmon.
4. Heat the almond butter in a small saucepan over medium heat.

5. Cook minced garlic
6. Drizzle the garlic-butter sauce over the salmon and asparagus and scatter the Parmesan cheese on top.
7. Bake in the preheated oven for about 12 minutes. You can switch the oven to broil at the end of cooking time for about 3 minutes to get a nice char on the asparagus.
8. Let cool for 5 minutes before serving.

Nutrition:

Calories 435,

26g fat,

42g protein

Lemon Rosemary Roasted Branzino

Preparation Time: 15 minutes
Cooking Time: 30 minutes
Servings: 2

Ingredients:

- 4 tablespoons extra-virgin olive oil, divided
- 2 (8-ounce) Branzino fillets
- 1 garlic clove, minced
- 1 bunch scallions
- 10 to 12 small cherry tomatoes, halved
- 1 large carrot, cut into ¼-inch rounds
- ½ cup dry white wine
- 2 tablespoons paprika
- 2 teaspoons kosher salt
- ½ tablespoon ground chili pepper
- 2 rosemary sprigs or 1 tablespoon dried rosemary
- 1 small lemon, thinly sliced
- ½ cup sliced pitted kalamata olives

Directions:

1. Heat a large ovenproof skillet over high heat until hot, about 2 minutes. Add 1 tablespoon of olive oil and heat
2. Add the Branzino fillets, skin-side up, and sear for 2 minutes. Flip the fillets and cook. Set aside.
3. Swirl 2 tablespoons of olive oil around the skillet to coat evenly. Add the garlic, scallions, tomatoes, and carrot, and sauté for 5 minutes Add the wine, stirring until all ingredients are well combined. Carefully place the fish over the sauce.
4. Preheat the oven to 450ºF (235ºC).
5. Brush the fillets with the remaining 1 tablespoon of olive oil and season with paprika, salt, and chili pepper. Top each fillet with a rosemary sprig and lemon slices. Scatter the olives over fish and around the skillet.
6. Roast for about 10 minutes until the lemon slices are browned. Serve hot.

Nutrition:

Calories 724, 43g fat, 57g protein

Grilled Lemon Pesto Salmon

Preparation Time: 5 minutes

Cooking Time: 10 minutes

Servings: 2

Ingredients:

- 10 ounces (283 g) salmon fillet
- 2 tablespoons prepared pesto sauce
- 1 large fresh lemon, sliced
- Cooking spray

Directions:

1. Preheat the grill to medium-high heat. Spray the grill grates with cooking spray.
2. Season the salmon well. Spread the pesto sauce on top.
3. Make a bed of fresh lemon slices about the same size as the salmon fillet on the hot grill, and place the salmon on top of the lemon slices. Put any additional lemon slices on top of the salmon.
4. Grill the salmon for 10 minutes.
5. Serve hot.

Nutrition:

Calories 316, 21g fat, 29g protein

Steamed Trout with Lemon Herb Crust

Preparation Time: 10 minutes
Cooking Time: 15 minutes
Servings: 2

Ingredients:

- 3 tablespoons olive oil
- 3 garlic cloves, chopped
- 2 tablespoons fresh lemon juice
- 1 tablespoon chopped fresh mint
- 1 tablespoon chopped fresh parsley
- ¼ teaspoon dried ground thyme
- 1 teaspoon sea salt
- 1 pound (454 g) fresh trout (2 pieces)
- 2 cups fish stock

Directions:

1. Blend olive oil, garlic, lemon juice, mint, parsley, thyme, and salt. Brush the marinade onto the fish.
2. Insert a trivet in the Pressure Pot. Fill in the fish stock and place the fish on the trivet.
3. Secure the lid. Select the Steam mode and set the cooking time for 15 minutes at High Pressure.

4. Once cooking is complete, do a quick pressure release. Carefully open the lid. Serve warm.

Nutrition:

Calories 477,

30g fat,

52g protein

Desserts

Crème Caramel

Preparation Time: 60 Minutes

Cooking Time: 60 Minutes

Servings: 12

Ingredients:

- 5 cups of whole milk
- 2 tsp vanilla extract
- 8 large egg yolks
- 4 large-sized eggs
- 2 cups sugar, divided
- ¼ cup 0f water

Directions:

1. Preheat the oven to 350°F
2. Heat the milk with medium heat wait for it to be scalded.
3. Mix 1 cup of sugar and eggs in a bowl and add it to the eggs.
4. With a nonstick pan on high heat, boil the water and remaining sugar. Do not stir, instead whirl the pan. When the sugar forms caramel, divide it into ramekins.

5. Divide the egg mixture into the ramekins and place in a baking pan. Increase water to the pan until it is half full. Bake for 30 minutes.
6. Remove the ramekins from the baking pan, cool, then refrigerate for at least 8 hours.
7. Serve.

Nutrition:

Calories: 110kcal

Carbs: 21g

Fat: 1g

Protein: 2g

Galaktoboureko

Preparation Time: 30 Minutes

Cooking Time: 90 Minutes

Servings: 12

Ingredients:

- 4 cups sugar, divided
- 1 tbsp. fresh lemon juice
- 1 cup of water
- 1 Tbsp. plus 1 ½ tsp grated lemon zest, divided into 10 cups
- Room temperature whole milk
- 1 cup plus 2 tbsps. unsalted butter, melted and divided into 2
- Tbsps. vanilla extract
- 7 large-sized eggs
- 1 cup of fine semolina
- 1 package phyllo, thawed and at room temperature

Directions:

1. Preheat oven to 350°F
2. Mix 2 cups of sugar, lemon juice, 1 ½ tsp of lemon zest, and water. Boil over medium heat. Set aside.

3. Mix the milk, 2 Tbsps. of butter, and vanilla in a pot and put-on medium heat. Remove from heat when milk is scalded
4. Mix the eggs and semolina in a bowl, then add the mixture to the scalded milk. Put the egg-milk mixture on medium heat. Stir until it forms a custard-like material.
5. Brush butter on each sheet then arrange all over the baking pan until everywhere is covered. Spread the custard on the bottom pile phyllo
6. Arrange the buttered phyllo all over the top of the custard until every inch is covered.
7. Bake for about 40 minutes. cover the top of the pie with all the prepared syrup. Serve.

Nutrition:

Calories: 393kcal; Carbs: 55g; Fat: 15g; Protein: 8g

Kourabiedes Almond Cookies

Preparation Time: 20 Minutes

Cooking Time: 50 Minutes

Servings: 20

Ingredients:

- 1 ½ cups unsalted butter, clarified, at room temperature
- 2 cups Confectioners' sugar, divided
- 1 large egg yolk
- 2 tbsps. brandy
- 1 1/2 tsp baking powder
- 1 tsp vanilla extract
- 5 cups all-purpose flour, sifted
- 1 cup roasted almonds, chopped

Directions:

1. Preheat the oven to 350°F
2. Thoroughly mix butter and ½ cup of sugar in a bowl. Add in the egg after a while. Create a brandy mixture by mixing the brandy and baking powder. Add the mixture to the egg, add vanilla, then keep beating until the ingredients are properly blended
3. Add flour and almonds to make a dough.

4. Roll the dough to form crescent shapes. You should be able to get about 40 pieces. Place the pieces on a baking sheet, then bake in the oven for 25 minutes.
5. Allow the cookies to cool, then coat them with the remaining confectioner's sugar.
6. Serve.

Nutrition:

Calories: 102kcal; Carbs: 10g; Fat: 7g; Protein: 2g

Ekmek Kataifi

Preparation Time: 30 Minutes

Cooking Time: 45 Minutes

Servings: 10

Ingredients:

- 1 cup of sugar
- 1 cup of water
- 2 (2-inch) strips lemon peel, pith removed
- 1 tbsp. fresh lemon juice
- ½ cup plus 1 tbsp. unsalted butter, melted
- ½ lbs. frozen kataifi pastry, thawed, at room temperature
- 2 ½ cups whole milk
- ½ tsp. ground mastiha
- 2 large eggs
- ¼ cup fine semolina
- 1 tsp. of cornstarch
- ¼ cup of sugar
- ½ cup sweetened coconut flakes
- 1 cup whipping cream
- 1 tsp. vanilla extract
- 1 tsp. powdered milk
- 3 tbsps. of confectioners' sugar

- ½ cup chopped unsalted pistachios

Directions:

1. Set the oven to 350°F. Grease the baking pan with 1. Tbsp of butter.
2. Put a pot on medium heat, then add water, sugar, lemon juice, lemon peel. Leave to boil for about 10 minutes. Reserve.
3. Untangle the kataifi, coat with the leftover butter, then place in the baking pan.
4. Mix the milk and mastiha, then place it on medium heat. Remove from heat when the milk is scalded, then cool the mixture.
5. Mix the eggs, cornstarch, semolina, and sugar in a bowl, stir thoroughly, then whisk the cooled milk mixture into the bowl.
6. Transfer the egg and milk mixture to a pot and place on heat. Wait for it to thicken like custard, then add the coconut flakes and cover it with a plastic wrap. Cool.
7. Spread the cooled custard-like material over the kataifi. Place in the refrigerator for at least 8 hours.
8. Strategically remove the kataifi from the pan with a knife. Take it away in such a way that the mold faces up.

9. Whip a cup of cream, add 1 tsp. vanilla, 1tsp. powdered milk, and 3 tbsps. Of sugar. Spread the mixture all over the custard, wait for it to harden, then flip and add the leftover cream mixture to the kataifi side.

10. Serve.

Nutrition:

Calories: 649kcal; Carbs: 37g; Fat: 52g; Protein: 11g

Revani Syrup Cake

Preparation Time: 30 Minutes

Cooking Time: 3 Hours

Servings: 24

Ingredients:

- 1 tbsp. unsalted butter
- 2 tbsps. all-purpose flour
- 1 cup ground rusk or bread crumbs
- 1 cup fine semolina flour
- ¾ cup ground toasted almonds
- 3 tsp baking powder
- 16 large eggs
- 2 tbsps. vanilla extract
- 3 cups of sugar, divided
- 3 cups of water
- 5 (2-inch) strips lemon peel, pith removed
- 3 tbsps. fresh lemon juice
- 1 oz of brandy

Directions:

1. Preheat the oven to 350°F. Grease the baking pan with 1 Tbsp. of butter and flour.
2. Mix the rusk, almonds, semolina, baking powder in a bowl.

3. In another bowl, mix the eggs, 1 cup of sugar, vanilla, and whisk with an electric mixer for about 5 minutes. Add the semolina mixture to the eggs and stir.
4. Pour the stirred batter into the greased baking pan and place in the preheated oven.
5. With the remaining sugar, lemon peels, and water make the syrup by boiling the mixture on medium heat. Add the lemon juice after 6 minutes, then cook for 3 minutes. Remove the lemon peels and set the syrup aside.
6. After the cake is done in the oven, spread the syrup over the cake.
7. Cut the cake as you please and serve.

Nutrition:

Calories: 348kcal; Carbs: 55g; Fat: 9g; Protein: 5g

Almonds and Oats Pudding

Preparation Time: 10 Minutes

Cooking Time: 15 Minutes

Servings: 4

Ingredients:

- 1 tablespoon lemon juice
- Zest of 1 lime
- 1 and ½ cups of almond milk
- 1 teaspoon almond extract
- ½ cup oats
- 2 tablespoons stevia
- ½ cup silver almonds, chopped

Directions:

1. In a pan, blend the almond milk plus the lime zest and the other ingredients, whisk, bring to a simmer and cook over medium heat for 15 minutes.
2. Split the mix into bowls then serve cold.

Nutrition:

Calories 174

Fat 12.1

Fiber 3.2

Carbs 3.9

Protein 4.8

Milk Chocolate Peanut Butter Cups

Preparation Time: 10 minutes, plus 1 hour to chill

Cooking Time: 5 minutes

Servings: 2

Ingredients:

- Cooking spray
- 12 ounces milk chocolate, broken into pieces
- 2 tablespoons coconut oil
- 12 teaspoons natural creamy peanut butter
- 1/8 Teaspoon sea salt

Directions:

1. Spray 12 mini-muffin liners with cooking spray, then place in an 8-by-8 dish.
2. In a small saucepan, bring a cup of water to a boil, then reduce heat to a simmer. Fit a heat-proof medium bowl on top of the saucepan to make a double boiler. Add the chocolate and coconut oil to the bowl, stirring gently with a wooden spoon until smooth, about 5 minutes.

3. Fill one-third of each muffin liner with melted chocolate, then 1 teaspoon of peanut butter, and top with melted chocolate.
4. Transfer the dish to the refrigerator and allow to set for at least 1 hour.

Nutrition:

Calories: 194

Total Fat: 12g

Saturated Fat: 7g

Protein: 3g

Carbohydrates: 21g

Fiber: 1g

Sodium: 66mg

www.ingramcontent.com/pod-product-compliance
Lightning Source LLC
Chambersburg PA
CBHW070735030426
42336CB00013B/1976